Translating the Language of the Newborn

Explaining those first few days of life

Nancy McGinty

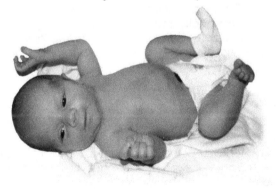

Waldenhouse Publishers, Inc.
Walden, Tennessee

Translating the Language of the Newborn

Thanks to the illustrators, Kay Tye Ogle and Jessie Claire McGinty for their generous contribution of the illustrations.

DISCLAIMER: Every baby and mother has individual needs. The information in this book is meant to be used as a guide. It, in no way, takes the place of information and instructions given to you by those medical professionals who are responsible for yours and your baby's care.

Published by Waldenhouse Publishers, Inc.
100 Clegg Street, Signal Mountain, Tennessee 37377 USA
888-222-8228 www,waldenhouse.com
ISBN: 978-1-947589-23-0
Library of Congress Control Number: 2019951432
   Describes behavior of the normal newborn infant in its first week
   of life and ways to attend to and manage its basic needs.
   – Provided by publisher
Printed in the United States of America

HEA041000	HEALTH & FITNESS / Pregnancy & Childbirth
HEA046000	HEALTH & FITNESS / Children's Health
HEA044000	HEALTH & FITNESS / Breastfeeding

To

All the wonderful newborns and their
parents who have taught me so much

Table of Contents

What Is My Newborn Telling Me?

As a neonatal nurse and lactation consultant, I have worked with thousands of newborns and their parents for thirty years. All of these parents want to know how to give their babies everything their little ones need. The big problem is that these newborns are not very good at using their words. These days, when parents hold their baby for the first time, it is likely the first time they have held a baby. They may have read a book or taken a class, but holding your own brand new baby is a life altering experience.

Babies are really very simple. They want to feel secure. They want to be warm and they want to eat when they are hungry. Parents, especially first time parents, don't speak baby. An important thing to remember is that you just met your baby and your baby has just met you. Be patient, you will get to know each other quickly. Your baby will stare at your face while you are staring at theirs. It won't be long before your baby associates your face with comfort and safety. It will be you who will make your baby the happiest. Meeting your baby's early, basic needs goes a long way to teach this little person to trust.

This is a short little book because it is only meant to cover your baby's first few days of life. This is a time when parents are exhausted and often overwhelmed with this new sense of responsibility. They hand you this baby and may tell you to feed this little person every three hours. You may get a quick lesson in cleaning and diapering and you're told to get some rest. If baby was delivered by c-section, or if the labor was long, then rest is what you need. There are so many things to consider that rest is hard to come by.

When your baby doesn't want to eat every three hours and when this is the first time you've changed a diaper, you wonder how you can take care of this precious baby. Combine this with parents who are exhausted or in pain and it can feel out of control.

Most hospitals have wonderful staff who are good at their jobs and really want to help. Sometimes new parents don't even know the questions to ask. If mother is breast feeding, ask for a lactation consultant if one does not routinely come to your room.

Babies don't plan. They work on instinct and reflex. They have several reflexes that are present at birth and then fade as the baby gets older. One of these that is most readily apparent to new parents is the suck reflex.

In the next pages, we will discuss these reflexes and the basic behavior and responses of the newborn baby from the baby's perspective.

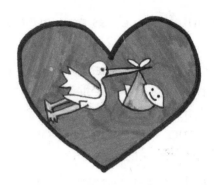

Why I Won't Wake Up

Labor is a very strenuous physical activity. Mommy and Daddy were probably exhausted after this workout. Labor for a first baby can last for several hours with a few hours of pushing. For people who are already sleep deprived this is mind numbing. Remember, I have been in labor just as long as Mommy has and I'm just as tired. My little body has had to make some pretty big adjustments. I am using my lungs for the first time and my liver is getting its first workout. So, I'm using energy for these two pretty important activities.

I was wide awake right after I was born because who wouldn't be wide awake with such a drastic change in surroundings? If allowed, I probably ate very well. I have been storing energy for the last several weeks. It's this energy that lets me stay awake right after birth and suck so strongly.

My stomach is about the size of a walnut holding about 1 to 2 teaspoons or 5 to 10 milliliters of formula or colostrum. If I get that much food at my first feeding, then I may sleep for several hours without getting hungry.

People tell Mommy to feed me every three hours. Well, I just might not be hungry every three hours, or I may be hungry again in thirty minutes. Please don't limit my feedings. Just like big people, my appetite can't be set by a clock. You probably want to offer me food every three hours because I may be sleeping so soundly that I forget about eating. Please don't tell me that I can't be hungry, because if I am breast feeding, no one but me knows how much I got at the last feeding. I only understand that I'm hungry or I'm not hungry. I'm sorry, Mommy, but I'm not old enough to be considerate of your time or your feelings yet.

I know, I know. You've heard "never wake a sleeping baby" but that just doesn't work when I am so brand new. I can go to sleep and sleep for six or more hours. This might be okay on my first day, but probably not on my second day. My blood sugar may drop too low and I can get a little dehydrated. Both of these things can make it even less likely that I'll wake up on my own.

I hate being unwrapped. I hate even more being naked. You can wake me up by making me a little uncomfortable. Don't keep me all snuggled up in a blanket in your arms. That's just an invitation for me to stay asleep. Take my blanket and shirt off and hold me out from your body. This will almost always get my attention.

If I am being fed by bottle, I will suck when the nipple touches the roof of my mouth, so this can wake me up. If I am breast feeding, I'm less likely to latch to a nipple while asleep. You can hand express some breast milk into a spoon and feed it to me. Remember, I'm a sucker not a sipper yet, so only give me a drop or two at a time with a spoon. These drops will probably wake me up, so latch me quickly to your breast.

Please don't let me go longer than three hours without eating after my first day. Colostrum or formula keep me well hydrated and help prevent jaundice. The more food I get, the more meconium I pass. This helps decrease problems with jaundice.

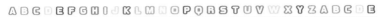

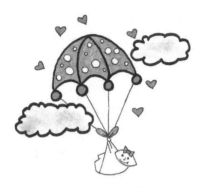

Why I Won't Eat

I know, I ate so well after I was born and now I won't even wake up, or if I'm awake, I won't eat. You've been told that I need to eat, so what's a mommy to do?

Some of the reasons I won't eat are very simple. Some are a little more complicated. If I ate very well at my first feeding, fifteen to twenty minutes or more at the breast or one half ounce of formula, then I might still be full. I may get as much as half an ounce of colostrum at that feeding. My tummy is small but will get bigger quickly. This is why colostrum increases gradually every day until mature milk is in and the amount of that increases daily. So, the reason I won't eat is that I may still be full. I won't breast feed unless I'm hungry.

Another reason that I have a problem eating is that I have forgotten how to suck. Sucking well right after birth is probably a survival tactic. It enables me to get that first good amount of energy supplying food.

Now, a nipple is in my mouth and I don't have any idea of what to do with it. I may have given strong feeding cues but still I won't suck. I need some help, please. My reflexes and instincts tell me to give feeding cues, and I'm hungry, but I don't know how to get the job done. If Mommy or Daddy will put their pinky finger in my mouth and keep it there while I try to figure out what to do, I will start to suck. Let me suck on your finger for several seconds and then quickly move me to the breast or bottle.

Another of my confounding activities is to latch on to Mommy's breast, suck twice and scream. I'm an instant gratification kind of guy or girl. Breasts don't give milk without being asked. This is a good thing and is called the let down phase. This let down reflex keeps mommy from walking around with a wet shirt all of the time.

I have to suck several times before I get any milk from the breast. My experience is limited and my patience is nonexistent. Hand expressing a few drops of colostrum or milk and letting me have it may be just the trick to give me some hope, and I'll latch on. If there isn't enough colostrum, a few drops of formula can accomplish the same thing.

Not eating in my first 24 hours is worrisome but not that unusual. If I'm a healthy normal newborn then this is okay. If I have a medical condition such as low blood sugar or jaundice that requires me to eat more on my first day, then ask my nurse or a lactation consultant to help you feed me.

If I've gone several hours, more than four, without eating, then I may just not realize I am hungry. Mommy can hand express a few drops and give them to me. If my eyes open and my hands go to my mouth, then you've reminded me of eating. If I continue to sleep and don't respond to the drops of food, then I'm not ready to eat. Keeping me skin to skin will encourage me to eat.

Please don't let me go longer than three hours, or four max, without eating after my first day, as that can cause problems with my weight and increase my risk for jaundice.

Mommies are often confused by what they think are conflicting instructions, but the fact is, Mommy and I are in dynamic states. The sleepy baby yesterday, day one, is the hungry, wide awake baby on day two. Mommy's breasts change every day. On my first day, I have extra fluid in my body and that is why nurses don't get so worried about my sparse eating that day. If I am spitting up amniotic fluid, I'm not going to want to eat until that leaves my body.

A B C D E F G H I J K L M N O P Q R S T U V W X Y Z A B C D E

So instructions for day one don't work for day two, three or four. Having more food will help push the meconium out of my body, lowering my risk for jaundice. So how mommies are asked to feed their babies depends on the age of the baby and his or her health conditions.

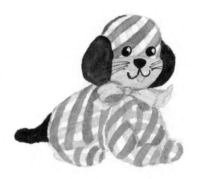

My Hands Are My Best Friends

While I was hanging around waiting to be born I had to entertain myself with whatever was closest to me. Most of the time this was my hands. I would hold on to my umbilical cord. I would touch my body and my face. The bond I formed with my hands remains after I am out in the big, exciting world. I still use my hands to explore this new place. Imagine touching cloth for the first time or touching Mommy's breast. When I touch things with my hands, my eyes can see the object and I begin to make connections.

I know that I have fingernails and everyone is so scared that I will scratch out my eyes. Well, I've had those fingernails and eyes for quite a few weeks and so far so good. It's rare that a baby hurts himself or herself with their fingernails. They make a baby emery board that you can file my nails with. Don't cut my nails because they are still attached to my skin.

I use my hands to help me realize when I am hungry. I may be half asleep, but if I put my hand in my mouth and start sucking, it gives me the idea to eat. Sucking my hands is one of the best indicators of how hungry I am. If I am really hungry, I'll have my fists balled and up to my face.

Just like my hands tell you when I'm hungry, they will also tell you when I'm full. When I'm hungry my hands are up to my face and my arms are tense. As I eat, my hands open and relax, signaling that I am getting full.

So, what I'm getting at, Mommy and Daddy, is please don't cover my hands. That would be like someone blindfolding you.

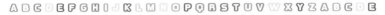
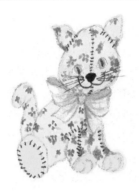

I Love to Suck
(on almost everything)

Sucking is one of the most important things that I do. It sounds so easy but that isn't always the case. I may have been sucking for many weeks before I was born. I had to suck on what was available. The most convenient thing was my tongue, then my lip, then my fingers. After I'm born, it's very important that I suck on Mommy's nipple or a bottle nipple.

This is where it can get so confusing. When offered the breast or bottle, I will continue to suck on whatever made me happy before I was born. This may interfere with my eating, so Mommy will need some help in teaching me to suck the right way.

Most of us babies will eagerly eat in our first hour of life. This birth process has been exhausting but also exciting. I am wide awake and I have all of the energy that I've stored up in the weeks before I was born. I will latch on to Mommy or a bottle and eat for up to 45 minutes. I have all that energy and Mommy has all of the colostrum she's been making for months. It's perfect. I get lots of colostrum and I have my first lesson in sucking for food.

Mommy is so happy and believes she has this feeding thing down. Surprise, surprise! When she wants to feed me again, I may have forgotten how to suck. I also could be so full that I don't want to eat again.

One way to find out is to put your pinky finger in my mouth. If I suck your finger then I will probably eat. You may find that my suck is more like biting, or that I don't make any effort to suck. If I'm biting, leave your finger in my mouth until I can figure out what to do. You can feel the change from bite to suck. If I won't suck at all, then I'm not hungry.

If my suck isn't strong then I probably can't get the colostrum out of the breast. Put your finger in my mouth and while I'm sucking, pull your finger out. If it's not hard to pull your finger out, then my suck may not be strong enough to get the job done. This is another time that finger sucking will help me and let me build strength in my tongue and cheeks.

Colostrum is thick and there's not much of it after the first big feeding. There's a reason for this. Sucking and swallowing takes coordination. I may need a little time to make this work. Colostrum's thickness and small amount make learning this task much easier. Colostrum is so rich in everything I need that a few drops can satisfy me and raise my blood sugar.

If I won't suck and you're worried about me, maybe one of those annoying people (nurse, lactation consultant) who keep coming into our room can show you how to hand express your milk and give it to me with a spoon. This little bit of colostrum on my tongue might be enough to encourage me to latch on and eat.

I will suck on anything. I will happily latch on to your nipple and suck for 30 minutes or more. I won't know that your nipple will be sore when I finish, and I'm too young to be concerned about that. It will be up to you, Mommy, to help me latch on the right way. The right way is to wait for me to open my mouth widely and then quickly, while supporting my head with your finger and thumb, push me deeply on to the breast and getting the nipple deeply in my mouth.

I have to squeeze the milk out of your breast, into your nipple and down my throat. If I'm sucking only on your nipple, I will flatten it, bruise it and eventually cause it to bleed. It's a good idea to have an experienced nurse or lactation consultant teach you how to get this good latch. Many new moms are afraid to push their baby firmly enough to get that good latch, so being shown is best.

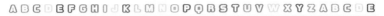

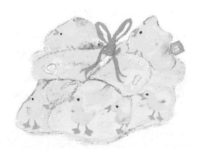

Dancing Chest to Chest
(Kangaroo Care)

I have spent the last months in a climate controlled home. It's the only place I've ever lived. I didn't have to eat or wear clothes or ask for anything. I got my food constantly. I could pee without a diaper. The main thing I could hear was Mommy's heartbeat. Of course, there were growls and gurgles from some place and some sounds that I really didn't understand.

I did like it when I could hear a noise that made Mommy dance. I loved it when we moved. It was always dark and I couldn't smell much. I did get the hiccups a lot but they really didn't bother me. There were certain times of the day and night that I liked to sleep or stay awake. I was pretty regular with these periods.

So now, I am transported to this strange new place. It's so bright. It's so loud and it's so cold. I have so much room to move and I don't like that. It doesn't feel right or safe. You can watch me and you'll see that I keep my arms and legs bent, and I don't stretch out.

Please, please take this silly shirt off me, and put me on my Mommy's chest. It's my perfect place to recover from the amazing journey I've just made. It's warm. I can hear that wonderful thump, thump of Mommy's heart that I've known for so long. I can smell now and my mommy smells so good. I even recognize her voice as that muffled noise I heard before.

If you can't put me back where I came from, then put me on Mommy's chest. When I get cool, and I am on Mommy's chest, Mommy's body warms up to regulate my temperature, and then when I am warmed up, Mommy's body cools down. How about that? Mommies are amazing. Daddies can put me skin to skin too, but without all that warming and cooling business. Just keep my back covered.

Now, this skin to skin thing sounds so simple and basic, but it has actually saved babies lives. Who knows how this all works, but it does work. I can be so upset and then be put on Mommy's chest and after a minute or so, I will calm right down. It

A B C D E F G H I J K L M N O P Q R S T U V W X Y Z A B C D E

takes a while for me to get so upset so it may take a while for me to calm down.

The sooner I am put on Mommy's chest after birth the better it is for me and for Mommy.

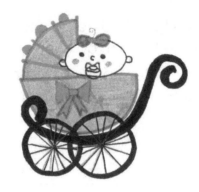

Now I want to eat
(all the time)

My second day of life comes quickly for Mommy but for me it's a lifetime. I've had time to rest up after the birth workout I went through. My tummy is empty and I'm getting hungry. I'm hard wired to eat. If given the opportunity I will usually get to work on the job of eating.

Remember, I am working on reflex and instinct. Even though I probably couldn't explain it, even if I could talk, I know that the more I nurse, the faster the breast milk will come in. If I'm getting formula, I will be able to go longer between feedings. If I'm breast feeding, Mommy's milk gradually increases until, usually by day 3 to day 5, I get enough to keep me happy for a couple of hours. I hear this is called cluster feeding. I will eat and then go to sleep. Mommy thinks I'm satisfied, but when she

A B C D E F G H I J K L M N O P Q R S T U V W X Y Z A B C D E

tries to lay me down, I wake up and demand to be fed again. If I am latched on properly, then this is all normal and will slow down when I get the milk supply to increase.

If my latch isn't deep enough, then I won't get very much milk when I eat. Mommy's nipple has more than one job. The nipple touching the roof of my mouth triggers my suck. The other job that the nipple does is act like a straw to let me get the milk from the breast. If I am clamping down on the tip of the nipple, I am "collapsing the straw" and the milk comes out in tiny amounts. That's why it is a really good idea to let one of those nurses or lactation consultants help you get me latched on the right way. The right way is to have the nipple as deep in my mouth as possible so I can squeeze the milk out of the breast and into the nipple.

So, if I am eating every hour and I am latched correctly, I am working to make Mommy's breast make more milk. This can be very tiring and worrisome for mommies because they think they are doing something wrong. If I'm not losing too much weight, and if I am having wet and poopy diapers, then I am doing okay.

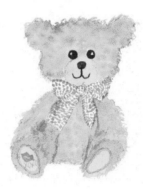

To Burp or Not to Burp

Burping is one of those things that confound parents. Does my baby need to be burped frequently or even at all? How do I hold my baby to burp, and how hard do I pat the back?

Burping is really an individual thing. One size does not fit all. If I have been crying while you changed my diaper and then you try to feed me, then yes, I may have swallowed a lot of air, and I won't want to eat until I get rid of that bubble of air.

If I'm breast feeding, I may not burp much, but if I am bottle feeding, I probably need to be burped more often. Until we get to know each other, please try to burp me frequently. Most of the time if I need to burp, I will just stop eating until I can burp. So, if I'm wide awake and lying there looking at you, please try to burp me and I can finish that feeding.

Another sign that I might need to be burped often is if I spit up. If I take milk on top of a big bubble of air, then air and milk will come back up in form of a spit up. Remember, we are still getting to know each other. If you've patted me on the back for five minutes and I haven't burped, then I probably don't need to.

The best way to hold me for burping is on your shoulder. Another way is to sit me on your lap and hold my head up by having your hand under my chin, not on my neck, please. Changing my position, such as rocking me back and forth, can also help me burp.

Burping can serve another purpose and that is to wake me up. When I get comfortable, I will go to sleep. When I eat, I'm happy and warm and being snuggled – a perfect invitation for a nap. Burping me gets my attention and brings me back to the task at hand.

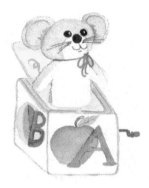

I'm Awake All Night

Days and nights mean nothing to me. My home for nine months had the same temperature, light, and taste. Of course there was more movement and more noise at times. Sometimes the noise and movement kept me awake, or it might have put me to sleep. Only Mommy knows the answer to this. The fact is that I am the same baby that I was before I was born.

If I was active and moving about during the day and getting quiet and sleeping at night, that will probably be the routine I follow on the outside. The only things that have changed for me are there is more room, noise, light and people. On the flip side, if I slept during the day but kept Mommy awake at night with my gymnastics, this is the routine I will have in the big bright world. It's important to keep a written record of every time

I eat, because if I am a night owl, I may eat four times during the night. If that's the case, I don't have to eat as many times during the day.

Some mommies are night people so a night owl baby is great, but if that schedule doesn't suit, then I can be changed. It can't be done quickly. I still have to eat 8-10 times a day, so Mommy will have to wake me up more during the day. Then at night if I am sleeping soundly when Mommy and Daddy are ready to go to bed, one of them should quietly get me up and feed me.

I would love to play at that time, but Mommy or Daddy cannot talk to me or sing or turn on too many lights. This is the time to do the job of eating and then sleeping. Hopefully, this will give Mommy and Daddy a longer period to sleep when it is dark.

I can sleep very soundly. A good way to gently wake me up is to take my clothes off. Please leave my diaper on. For some reason, when I poop or pee on big people it upsets them. Actually, changing my diaper is a good way to get my attention.

Of course, as soon as I get close to my wonderful mommy's body, I may go right back to sleep. Like I mentioned before, skin to skin is a good way to get me to wake and eat. I may sleep there for a little while, but if I can find my hand to suck on, I'll wake myself up.

My last accommodations were a bit tight, so I kept my legs bent and my arms close to my body. Gently stretching me out can make me a little uncomfortable and I'll wake up.

We babies eat when we're hungry and sleep when we're sleepy. It really is all about us, for a little while anyway.

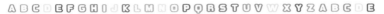

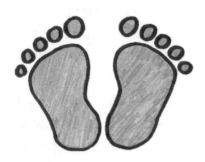

I'm Changing Quickly

On my first day, I was so tired. All that I wanted to do was sleep and maybe eat a little. By day two, I was beginning to wake up but still wanted to sleep most of the time. Now by day three I am doing better with eating, and now if I'm breast feeding, I want to eat all of the time. This is called cluster feeding and is okay if I have a good latch. As mentioned earlier in the book, Mommies can get confused because they are told one thing on day one and something different on days two and three.

The reason for this is because Mommy and I are in dynamic states. Mommy's body is changing rapidly, and I am changing fast too. Waking up and mastering this eating thing are big deals for a first timer. Instructions for day one don't work for subsequent days. If you are giving me less than one ounce of formula on my first day, the amount needs to increase with every day of my life. Mommy's colostrum increases daily until I get lots of milk.

Please don't tell me I can't be hungry if I just ate but want to eat again, because I can. I really don't understand that other people have lives. Everything is all about me. I want to eat and I suck for five minutes and then get comfortable and go to sleep. Mommy may have other things to do, but for me, I'm happy with the way things are. Mommy and I will get this all worked out, but it will take several days.

I'll wake up more each day. I will begin to set eating and sleeping patterns. Please don't try to schedule me for about three to four weeks. It takes us about that long to get settled in with each other.

~ ~ ~

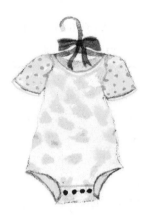

It's Going to be Okay

As a nurse, I can't remember meeting a first time mother or father who wasn't scared of caring for their new baby. Fear and guilt are the difficult parts of parenting, and yet, they do serve a purpose. They make us hyper vigilant. They make us pay attention to our babies' needs.

There are really only two things a new parent has to do. The first and most important is to feed the baby. Babies need fuel to operate just like older children do. Breast milk is best but by no means the only way to feed your baby. For some babies, the small amount of colostrum at first is not enough to satisfy them. These babies will breast feed for thirty minutes on each breast and still cry and suck vigorously on their hands. This baby is still hungry. It is not true that giving this baby a small amount of formula will ruin breast feeding. If your baby is telling you he or she is very hungry, it is the parent's responsibility to feed that baby.

The second thing a parent has to do is keep your baby clean and warm. It really is this simple in these early days. In one culture, a new mother is put in a small hut with her newborn. She is given everything she needs to be comfortable and well fed. She stays there for forty days and then she emerges and introduces her baby to the village. It takes about forty days for things to settle down after a birth.

If mother is breast feeding, then she must pump or feed her baby 8 to 10 times a day. Breasts are very cooperative. They give as much or as little as they are asked to give. If breasts are not stimulated, then milk will dry up. If mother is feeding formula and using the powdered form, read the directions carefully and make sure you are mixing it correctly for a baby the age of yours.

Don't rely on Dr. Google for your information. There are reliable websites that reference their work and list their sources. Be suspicious of websites that make you feel frightened or guilty. Make notes of questions to ask your pediatrician or lactation consultant. Find a peer group of like minded mothers. There are few problems that have not been experienced and solved by someone.

Like millions of parents before you, you will be great parents. Common sense will get you through most situations. You'll gain confidence every day. Feed your baby, protect your milk supply, if that is important to you, and the rest will fall into place.

.

Century Gothic and Colourbars on LSI 50# archival white
Type and design by Karen Paul Stone

To order additional copies of

Translating
the Language of the Newborn

Please copy this page, complete the information,
and mail with check or money order to
Nancy McGinty, 74 Sam Allen Mountain Road, Ellijay, GA 30536
OR
Visit http://www.translatingthelanguageofthenewborn.com

Name _____

Shipping address _____

_____

City _____ State ____ Zip _____

Phone _____

E-mail (optional for order confirmation)

_____

Quantity ____ @ $12.95   = $ _____

Shipping first book @ $4.85   = $ _____

Ship additional books @ $3.00   = $ _____

                        Subtotal   = $ _____

GA residents add sales tax @ 7% = $ _____

                        TOTAL = $ _____

**Please copy this page, complete the information,
and mail with check or money order to
Nancy McGinty, 74 Sam Allen Mountain Rd, Ellijay, GA 30536
OR
Visit http://www.translatingthelanguageofthenewborn.com**